BULLY PROOF FITNESS

The ultimate guide for parents to win the battle against bullies, bellies and make your kid feel like a super ninja!

By Chris Casamassa
#1 Bestselling Author

Table of Contents

Welcome to BULLY PROOF FITNESS!

This book represents nearly thirty years of hard work, experience and the efforts of my incredible team and customers. You may well be one of them!

Here is what you can to expect in this book, so you will get the most out of it and your expectations are met.

First, it's interactive. There are lots of opportunities for you to go deeper into the content, gain access to free training videos, or participate in some free interactive events and bonus training. Our goal is to help and empower 1,000,000 kids to be fitter, more confident and more bully proof than ever before.

Second, this book is for parents and school administrators. It's intended to help your child become more physically fit, more confident and more self-assured than ever before.

Third, it's for gyms, day care centers, fitness camps, boot camps, personal trainers, martial arts schools, instructors and anyone – any*where* – that works with, trains, guides, empowers or teaches kids to become the best possible versions of themselves as they develop into full-grown adults. You'll find a *lot* of ideas that you can use to grow your business, in almost any industry, country or language, anywhere in the world.

If you're looking for free, easy money, this isn't the book for you. I'm not here to blow smoke up your butt and lie to you. Working with kids is difficult at times but it's rewarding – both spiritually and financially – if it's done right!

Fourth, this book wasn't intended to be a NY Times #1 Bestseller (though that would be nice.) It's designed to start a conversation with you; to give you and me a chance to get to know each other better, develop trust and a bond, and ultimately help us to decide if we can help your child or the kids in your community get fit, strong, confident and healthy by working together.

Fifth, this is a book that's short, but packed with implementable content – as well as lots of ideas. My intention, and the purpose of this book, is to show you the most powerful ways to help children (and their parents) reduce the risk of bullying, prevent their child from ever *becoming* a bully, ease stress, get stronger and leaner while they lose weight, and raise their self esteem. Our goal is to help build confidence all while increasing a child's overall academic GPA. We have a how-to system available that includes everything you need to execute what you'll read in these pages.

You'll notice there are opportunities throughout this book to watch some free training videos – and YES, I do have some great products that you can invest in; products that will help us reach our goal of impacting 1,000,000 kids on their path to being Bully Proof. For parents, we offer 'at home training programs as well as licensed training facilities all around the country. Please visit www.kicknfitkids.com locations to find your closest center.

If you are a small business owner, we have licensing opportunities available. Our done-for-you model shows and teaches you exactly how to run a successful, confidence-building program for kids through step-by-step instructions. Our license program is secured by zip code and complete license info is available at www.businesskombat.com join our team of over 100 certified licensed locations. Our system of helping kids is proven, and it works fast.

Having said that, if you like what you read, or at least *most* of what you read, I'd absolutely, positively love to hear from you, get to know you better, and have you post a success story, picture or video and comment on my Facebook wall. You can find me on almost any social media channel. Just type in my name, or the name of this book.

The BEST way to start a relationship with me, and get all the information you need, is to visit the web links in this book. Join me for the free training, and learn more about how to help kids have fun, get fit and be healthy. It's my privilege and honor to help kids, parents, families and communities change their lives for the better, and keep kids on the journey to being Bully Proof and fit!

Respectfully
Chris Casamassa, Glendora, California, USA

PS - if you love this book, or your child feels better because of it, would you please post a review on Amazon? If you DON'T like it, send me an email, social@reddragonkarate.com explaining why and I'll give you a full refund. How does that sound?

Please be kind. I have kids too. They read what people say about me online, and so do their friends. There's no sense in dragging innocent kids into something unnecessary. Nobody likes a bully, and our world has too much hate in it already. Let's be friends. Cool?

PPS – I'm going to repeat myself – if you enjoy this book or found it useful, I'd be very grateful if you posted a short review on Amazon. Your support makes a difference and I read all the reviews personally so I can make this book even better.

Thanks again for your support.

Now, let's get to work making your kids Bully Proof!

Endorsements and Accolades

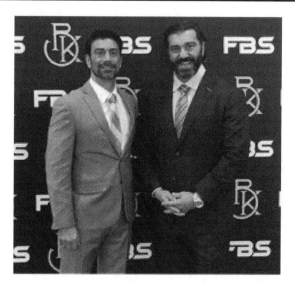

"Chris never ceases to amaze me with his ability to connect with people, and make it easy and fun to learn how to handle bullies. He may play the role of a super hero in movies, but he truly is a hero for kids and adults who have ever been bullied. Learn from his expertise and watch your kids become bully proof!"

**Bedros Keuilian,
Founder of Fit Body Boot Camp**

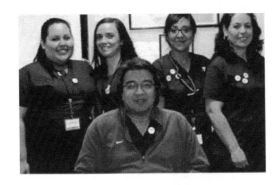

I have been a practicing family medicine for over 30 years. Since meeting Chris in the 90's I have witnessed first hand how he has made a difference in our younger generation with his teachings. As a Martial arts professional, he has demonstrated to me that he is a thorough, caring and intelligent professional.

His knowledge and insights in getting kids Bully Proof and fit are without equal. Kids need to be fit. In addition to benefiting their general health, it also makes their mind stronger and more confident. I highly recommend his teachings and the advise in this book.

Dr. Cris Armada, Jr., DO
Armada Wellness & Family Care

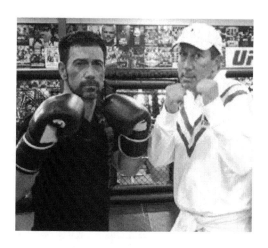

"Chris Casamassa is the country's champion, as a 4 time #1 North American Sport Karate competitor. Chris is *my* champion, because he plays Scorpion in all the *Mortal Kombat* movies and TV shows I produce.

But these things are not what really convinced me Chris is a champion, in the true sense of the word. Something else did. Here's the story.

We had a launch party for the first *Mortal Kombat* movie. One aspiring martial artist/wanna be actor cornered Chris and rambled on and on, bragging about how he could kick anyone's butt, his style was the best and he was the toughest guy there.

Now this guy had no idea who Chris was. Neither guy had any idea I was listening. By the way, Chris could have killed him in like 15 seconds.

But Chris did not tell him that. He did not brag. He did not interrupt. He did not point out the ridiculous nature of all the things the wannabe tough guy talked about. He did not embarrass the guy as he easily could have.
Chris politely stood there, listened, nodded and simply let the guy finish. Then he moved on.

Then I *knew* that Chris is a real champion. One who knows it and doesn't have to prove it to every insecure dude out there.He's a real champ who doesn't need to show off and lets his actions speak, not his words.

From that moment on, Chris and I have been friends. He's been in lots of our productions. He hosts a really popular show on our network, Blackbelt TV. He is slated to play a lead in one of our upcoming movies.

He is always, *always* enthusiastic, full of ideas and creative ways to help and make things better.

Chris doesn't even interrupt me in public when I tell everyone I taught him everything he knows about martial arts (which is 100% not true, of course). In all seriousness, we do something on all our sets with Chris called 'Move of the Day', where Chris teaches me one move each day. I've learned a ton from him, and this is now a feature on Blackbelt TV.

To find someone in the movie business talented in martial arts and acting is rare. To find someone like that who is also classy, humble and helpful – as Chris is – is almost impossible. So here's the deal. This book will help your kids. This book will help the world, because bullying sucks and he can help negate it.

If you are a business owner, this book will help you make money. But here is the surprise – this book will also help you, no matter who you are, because learning from the mind and soul of a true champion – of which there are precious few in the world – is priceless.

Larry Kasanoff
CEO of Threshold Entertainment

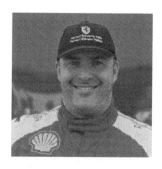

We are in the middle of perhaps the greatest health epidemic since the black plague. The adoption of the "western diet" combined with extremely low levels of activity have created the perfect obesity storm and the front line for this fight is our children. For us to turn the tide on this storm we need to educate and inspire our kids to take care of themselves, to exercise, and to take responsibility for their own health.

To lead this charge, we need people like Chris Casamassa. Chris has been on the front lines in the fight for our kids virtually his entire life. Whether teaching martial arts, conducting anti-bullying initiatives, helping to build kids self-confidence, or teaching self-discipline, Chris is uniquely qualified to rescue our kids. With this book Chris takes his lifetime of experience and channels it into a simple, effective, and fun program that your kids will love!

Jon Becker
Executive Director
The Becker Family Foundation

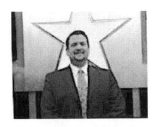

These days, it's hard to find leaders – in business and life – that actually walk the talk that they preach, Chris Casamassa, however, is one of those people. Chris and I met about 10 years ago when our kids started preschool together. Soon after, my wife and I decided to sign our kids up for a karate program at Chris's school. Upon entering the school I was immediately struck by the words that surrounded the Dojo, words like attitude, confidence, respect, focus, and quality. These are words that are easy to write on a wall, but hard to abide by.

After my kids spent nearly three years at Red Dragon Karate, I was convinced that Chris lived and breathed these words in both his professional and personal life. I have also witnessed him teach numerous bully proofing classes at our children's school – classes that have helped and inspired endless students and teachers to recognize and properly respond to bullies.

In my line of work, I am responsible for a Fortune 500 franchise business with an operations team built towards personal improvement and operational development, all while managing franchisee relationships.

I continue to live and lead by many of those words that I read on the walls of the Red Dragon Dojo. This is why I am proud to call Chris my friend, and feel that he is truly a person you and your kids can learn from

Daniel Boose
COO Friendly Franchisees Corporation

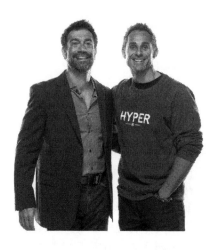

"Chris Casamassa is an amazing martial artist and trainer. He understands what it takes to inspire and educate today's youth to be great. Use the knowledge from this book to help motivate your family and change your community forever. If you own or operate a martial arts studio or gym, get his programs to help kids in your community get fit, strong and healthy while you grow your business"

Roland Osborne
Creator – Hyper Martial Arts

FREE - Bonus Training

This book includes access to **step-by-step training** you can use RIGHT NOW to help your kids get fit & Bully Proof in **just 5 minutes a day**!

No experience required!
Get it NOW at www.bullyprooffitness.com

Overview and Explanation

First, let's start with the definition of bullying:

verb present participle: bullying

1   use superior strength or influence to intimidate (someone), typically to force him or her to do what one wants: "a local man was bullied into helping them"

2   *synonyms*: persecute, oppress, tyrannize, browbeat, harass, torment, intimidate, strong-arm, dominate; *More informal* – push around, bullyrag.
    "The others bully him"

3   coerce, pressure, pressurize, press, push; force, compel; badger, goad, prod, browbeat, intimidate, dragoon, strong-arm.

    Informal - bulldoze, railroad, lean on

    "She was bullied into helping"

This book is not going to spend much time identifying and understanding the behaviors of bullies. There are dozens of books on that topic on the shelves already. You picked up this book for a reason – you, or someone you love, is currently or has been the victim of bullying.

This book is designed to STOP bullying, and to prevent you or your child from becoming one. If you or your child have some of the traits of a bully as outlined, we will show you how to "course correct" yourself to stop.

Wrong Way on a 1-Way Street

Psychologists are wrong.

School administrators are wrong.

Parents come to the wrong conclusions as to why their kids are being bullied.

Parents think that it reflects on them, and they sometimes blame themselves – this, too, is wrong. Parents should *never* blame themselves. There's a fundamental issue, and it's not what the psychologists say. It's not what the school system says. It's not what the parents think.

Here is what a bully looks for, plain and simple.

Weakness.

Yup, that's it. Bullies are like a pack of lions that spot a pride of gazelles. These predators don't pick a target at random – instead, they look for the smallest, easiest prey they can find. What is that lion looking for? Weakness. When they identify their target, they think, "that's the one. I'm gonna kill and eat *that* one"

Why didn't it pick the leader, standing up front, or the biggest gazelle in the middle? They chose the weakest, slowest and easiest one to grab.

Now, weakness can come in many forms. There is the obvious weakness that comes from an absence of physical strength, followed by weakness of self-confidence or self-esteem – and even weakness of character.

These weakness markers are what the bully sees as signals to attack. This happens daily to thousands of kids and adults all over the world, and there is a certain reason why these flaws are being targeted – they make for easy prey.

Our company, Lou Casamassa's Red Dragon Karate, has seen this trend and pattern tens of thousands of times over the last fifty years. Our students, as they come through our fourteen Red Dragon Karate Schools, come to learn that bullies and bad guys follow a very predictable pattern. They pick a potential victim, looking for the indicators that will help assure them that they have made the right choice.

Then there is a solution the psychologists, doctors, school systems and so-called "experts" won't address, - but we will within the pages of this book.

Now, I'm gonna stop you – before you say it, the answer is *not*, "punch the bully in the face". Although we *will* discuss and explore those options, violence can create more problems than it's worth. We want all kids and adults to be prepared, and to be confident in themselves. Most of all, we want people to walk away from – not into – a dangerous situation with their held high and their ego intact.

BULLY PROOF FITNESS uses a combination of short and simple training sessions, lasting 1-5 minutes, which can be tailored to any child or adult. With our easy to follow videos and guides kids can get fit, strong and healthy in no time!

This is the best system in the world to help kids get on track for success in school and life. Use this strategy along with the **BULLY PROOF FITNESS** bonuses that are included by heading to this link

www.bullyprooffitness.com

First thing's first, though. Who is Chris Casamasa, and why should you listen to or trust me?

I've been teaching, training, coaching and inspiring children since I was just a kid myself. I grew up in the martial arts, and got my start at 4 years old. Since I was 15 I've been teaching kids of all ages full-time as my hobby and my passion.

I've helped and guided over 50,000 students (kids and adults) during the past 35 years. These students have trained with me by attending one of our Red Dragon Studios workshops, training seminars or special events. I am now a 9th degree Black Belt, and the current President of the 14 Red Dragon Karate studios in southern California. I directly oversee operations, and help studio owners grow their business by focusing on two simple and important concepts – quality and service. With our programs – Lou Casamassa's Red Dragon Karate, KICKNFIT KIDS, The Kicknfit Challenge, B90Z Birthday success systems and now **BULLY PROOF FITNESS** – I have the honor and privilege of training, motivating, educating and inspiring over 400 school owners, instructors, personal trainers and managers on a weekly basis. I have also been fortunate enough to help tens of thousands of Martial Art students achieve their goals.

It is my honor and privilege to have the ability to speak, teach, train and inspire students and school owners around the globe, sharing ways that they can empower their students and supercharge their business.

I think it's reasonable to say that, over the course of my career, I have performed, taught, trained, instructed and coached tens of thousand of students on how to overcome their fears, grow stronger and more confident, live an empowered life and be able to stand tall in the face of adversity.

What excites me most is seeing the, "a-ha!" moment in a student's eyes when everything clicks into place. This is the moment that fear and doubt disappear, and a new, more confident and stronger person emerges. One who has the ability to walk without the fear they used to hold onto, and without the doubt and uncertainty of how to handle the challenges they face. Perhaps most importantly, they have the strength in both mind and body to be able to be bully proof! *That's* what this book and companion videos are all about.

I also competed professionally on the North American Sport Karate Tour (NASKA), where I became a 4 time #1 national champion. I have had the opportunity to appear in dozens of films and Television shows. I have doubled for George Clooney in *Batman & Robin*, appeared with Wesley Snipes in *Blade,* fought Chuck Norris in *Walker: Texas Ranger,* slayed vampires with *Buffy, **and so much more. My current mission is to help 1 million kids become BULLY PROOF!***

What is BULLY PROOF FITNESS, and how will it change the way Kids deal with bullies?

Because every kid needs something slightly different, and we want to get results as quickly as possible, how many of these traits sound familiar when it comes to your children?

- They don't have a ton of friends
- They don't have lots of energy
- They have lower grades than you would like
- They don't know how to express themselves when upset or sad
- They don't have good tempers
- They spend more time watching TV and on their video game consoles than playing outside
- They lack motivation

BULLY PROOF FITNESS is the solution for all of these challenges. With this program, you can:

- Start gaining new friends with similar interests
- Improve your children's grades, and their GPA
- This book includes step-by-step action plans you can implement with any kid
- There is no special equipment to buy
- There are no special pills, potions or fancy fad diets to follow

You can use our program to help kids of any fitness level. Even if they have never done sports or training of any kind!

Yes, Even I Was Bullied

Today, I am a 9th-degree Black belt, a four-time national champion, a celebrity motivational speaker and a movie star. It wasn't always like that, though – believe it or not, I was bullied as a kid. Here's my story.

When I was in junior high school, I was very short for my age. Of course, all of my friends started to grow much sooner and much faster, In fact, I was a very late bloomer. When I was in 7th grade I was only three feet eleven inches tall!

I had friends at the time who were four and a half feet, five feet tall when we got to eighth grade. Some of my friends shot all the way to almost six feet. Being the littlest guy in the room led to me getting picked on quite a bit, and thank goodness I had already been training and knew martial arts. That saved me from going into a shell and having a complete meltdown.

Now, at this time I was also a little chunky because I hadn't grown. Naturally, kids being the mean little bastards they can be, would pick on me and make fun of me because I was short and a little plump. One of my supposed friend's favorite things to call me was an Oompa Loompa. Again, my mental discipline from the martial arts training is what helped me and carried me through those times. It didn't stop people from picking on me, but it *did* allow me to have enough self-confidence and self-esteem to know that things would get better. Later I would be very thankful for that, though obviously I wasn't very happy at the time – nobody likes being picked on, even kids that grow up to play Batman.

So, as we've established, I was a late bloomer; I really didn't reach my full height until my senior year of high school. I was only 3 feet 11 inches tall as a sixth and seventh grader, I grew about three more inches when I got to eighth grade and I kind of stayed there, just a little over five feet tall, until I finally went through a giant growth spurt in the summer of my junior year of high school.

That made my junior high and early high school years pretty interesting. Again and again, I go back to the one thing that saved me both mentally and physically – my martial arts training.

When I got into high school, the upper classmen did a lot of hazing, which was pretty common. In our high school, one of the many things that the seniors liked to do to the freshman was to try and pick them up and put them in trash cans. Of course, on my third day of high school, this almost happened to me – though they didn't quite make it because I had enough skill to escape. I didn't fight them or hit them, but I did run and get away. Escape and defense were lessons learned from my martial arts training, so again, I was very thankful for that.

The attempted hazings continued – not just on me, but on many freshmen. One day I decided I wanted to try out for the wrestling team. Red Dragon Karate, which our style of martial arts, is a form of MMA that incorporates judo, a Japanese discipline known for its great throwing, ground holds and take downs, so I figured that wrestling was right up my alley.

The biggest guy on our wrestling team was a real heavyweight. He was a senior named Brian, and I remember him and the incident I'm about to describe to this day. This was the day that the bullying stopped, purely accidentally. Word got out on the wrestling team that I was in the martial arts and that I knew karate, which at the time was still a mystery to most Americans. This was well before *Ninja Turtles*, *Power Rangers* or *Mortal Kombat* were part of the pop culture landscape

Anyway, our senior heavyweight wrestler decided he was going to try and see what this little karate kid could do. I actually don't know what his intent was, but clearly he wanted me to show everybody that I either knew martial arts or I didn't. People had talked about how my Dad owned the local karate school in our town, so he put two and two together and figured out the name was the same. He asked me to do a kick, but I didn't want to – one of the first things we learn in the martial arts is to not show off or showcase our skill. Besides, I was still pretty shy and nervous; this was my first day out on the wrestling mats in the gym.

Brian kept goading me. "Just show me a kick, show me a kick, show me a kick," was seemingly all he could say. All the other wrestlers on the team were there – juniors, seniors, freshmen and sophomores – because it was day one orientation. I eventually agreed, if only to stop him running his mouth.

Now, Brian was six feet two inches tall, and at this time I was just a little over four feet. He held up his hand as high as his head and explained that he wanted me to kick it. I decided upon a roundhouse kick, which was at the time one of my favorite moves. He held up his hand and I said, "Okay, I'll do this and then you've got to leave me alone."

I went to do the kick, but unfortunately he was holding his hand very close to his face. You can probably guess where this story is leading – I missed my target. It got as high as his outstretched hand, but my kick landed directly on his cheek, making a clapping sound that seemed to echo around the entire gym – especially seeing as the place became deathly quiet. I thought he was going to kill me!

Instead, Brian looked at me, smiled, rubbed his cheek a little and said, "that was a good kick!" From that day we became friends and he kind of took me under his wing. What's more, something else happened in that moment – pretty much all the bullying stopped. Maybe that was because I gained the respect of the biggest, strongest guy in the school - albeit completely by accident. I never set out to do it, and I was scared as hell when I kicked that guy in the face. I had no interest in using mtraining to hurt people then, and I still don't today.

Again though, whether you're a martial artist or not, bullying can happen to anyone, anywhere, at any time. I just happened to be in a position and a place in my life where things worked out for me by chance. It doesn't always work like that for everybody and I don't recommend trying to kick the biggest, toughest guy at your school in the face! Remember, I set out to not do that – it was an accident that fortunately worked out in my favor.

The Bullying Epidemic

Real research into bullying yields some unreal results.

The following pages of real medical and scientific research offer just a small glimpse into the damaging effects of bullying. It also shows very conclusively that regular exercise has a *major* impact in helping kids of all ages adapt, react, respond and overcome the short and long term damage that bullying can do to their bodies.

The top three reasons for being bullied that are reported most often by school-aged students are looks (55%), body shape (37%), and race (16%) *(Davis & Nixon, 2010)*

The study results:

92% of kids who report being bullied report that it is because of their body shape and their looks.

Here's the thing – *it's not getting any better.*

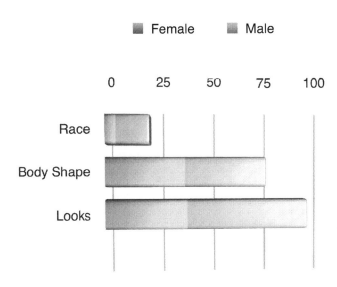

Despite a dramatic increase in public awareness and anti-bullying legislation nationwide, the prevalence of bullying is still one of the most pressing issues facing our nation's youth. It is one of our driving forces for writing this book, so that we can do everything in our power to get knowledge and information into the hands of parents and educators. Only as a community can we end the cycle of bullying, and the epidemic of childhood obesity.

In a study by the National Center for Educational Statistics in 2016, more than one out of every five students reported being bullied. Bullying affects individuals across ethnicity, gender, grade, and economic status, whether kids live in urban, suburban, or rural communities. Bullying can have serious effects during school years and well into adulthood.

In a study by Petrosino, Guckenburg, DeVoe, and Hanson, 64% of children who were bullied did not report it. *Only 36% reported the bullying.*

In a study by Hawkins, Pepler, and Craig, more than half of bullying situations, 57%, stop when a peer intervenes on behalf of the student being bullied.

In a study by Davis and Nixon in 2010, the reasons for being bullied reported most often by students were looks 55%, body shape 37%, and race 16%. **That means that 92% of bullying that students reported were based on their body shape and their looks.** If there's any more reason for your kids to be fit, confident strong and healthy, it's that right there.

There are dozens of mental and physical effects of bullying. Some of these include students who are at an increased risk of poor school adjustment, difficulty sleeping, and anxiety or depression. Students who *engage* in bullying behavior are at increased risk for academic problems, substance use, and violent behavior.

Students who are both targets of bullying *and* engage in bullying behavior are at a greater risk for both mental health and behavior health problems than students who only bully or are only bullied. Students who experience bullying are twice as likely as non-bullied peers to experience negative health effects such as headaches and stomachaches. Kids who self-blame and conclude they *deserve* to be bullied are more likely to face negative outcomes, such as depression, prolonged victimization, and maladjustments.

Now, here's another terrible number – 160,000.

It is estimated that **160,000 children** miss school *every day* due to fear of attack or intimidation by other students (*Source – National Education Association. American schools harbor approximately 2.1 million bullies and 2.7 million of their victims.*). Across the USA, nearly 20% of students report being bullied on school property.

Bullying is associated with academic struggle, low self-esteem, anxiety, depression, substance abuse, and self-harm. Exercise, conversely, has been widely reported to have robust positive effects on mental health including reduction in depression, anxiety, and substance abuse.

A group of researchers led by Dr. Jeremy Sibold of the University of Vermont examined the relationship between exercise frequency, sadness, and suicidal thoughts and attempts in 13,583 U.S. adolescents.

30% of students studied reported sadness for 2 or more weeks after being bullied; 22.2% and 8.2% reported suicidal thoughts and suicidal attempts in the same time period. Bullied students were twice as likely to report sadness, and three times as likely to report suicidal thoughts or attempt when compared to peers who were not bullied.

How Exercise Helps With Bullying

In an article taken from the website The Science of Us, Jesse Singal_points out that a great deal of research points to the physical and psychological benefits of exercise. These benefits are particularly important for teens, given that adolescence is a time of accelerated development and habit formation.

It's also, unfortunately, a time that a lot of kids get bullied.

A team led by Dr. Jeremy Sibold of the University of Vermont set out to investigate the correlation between exercise and bullying in their study, published in the Journal of the American Academy of Child & Adolescent Psychiatry. Overall, they found:

"25.1% of students who reported exercising on 6 to 7 days per week felt sad for 2 weeks or more in the past 12 months, compared to 35.7% of students who reported exercising on 0 to 1 day. Of students who exercised on 6 to 7 days in the past week, 15.9% reported suicidal ideation, and 6.4% reported suicide attempt in the past 12 months, compared to 24.6% and 10.3% of students who exercised on 0 to 1 day, respectively."

The benefits of exercise held, both for students who were bullied and those who weren't:

Taken together, these results certainly point to the idea that exercise can help prevent the worst psychological damage of bullying from really taking root. It's natural to expect, after all, that kids who exercise a lot are in better shape and, depending on the form of exercise, they may have an easier time finding other kids to hang out with.

Both of these might help prevent them from being victimized – or at least reduce the frequency and severity of victimization. This is especially important as being bullied leaves an imprint on a kid's brains. A new study from Children's Hospital Los Angeles and the University of Southern California, published on NYMag.com, examined the brains of bullying victims, and the results were not good.

The researchers tracked 83 kids from ages 9 to 14, both scanning their brains and asking them questions about their social lives and everyday stresses. The ability to process emotions and react to stress was larger in volume among 14-year-olds who had been bullied as children. In addition, previously bullied adolescents had thinner temporal and prefrontal cortexes, areas critical for processing information and regulating behavior. This thinning was seen in both sexes,

Here's the good news – *it can get better.*

Fact: Exercise on 4 or more days per week was associated with a startling 23% reduction in sadness, suicidal thoughts, and suicidal attempts in all bullied students.

Bullying is a severe and growing public health burden, with consequences reported across the lifespan. As a result, there is the possibility of exercise programs being seen as a public health approach to reduce suicidal behavior in all adolescents. This is a particularly important consideration, due to the fact that *many high schools in our country have little or no exercise programs for non-varsity athletes.*

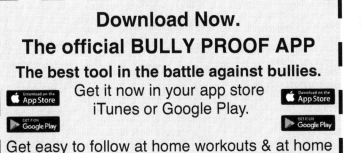
Source: The article "Physical Activity, Sadness, and Suicidality in Bullied US Adolescents" by Jeremy Sibold, Erika Edwards, Dianna Murray-Close, and James J. Hudziak (http://dx.doi.org/10.1016/j.jaac. 2015.06.019) appears in the Journal of the American Academy of Child and Adolescent Psychiatry, Volume 54, Issue 10 (October 2015), published by Elsevier.

Physical Fitness improves School Performance in Middle School Girls

In a 2016 study by Jamie Anne Donnelly at Walden University, found a direct relationship between physical fitness and school performance in middle school girls. The findings of her study confirmed the results of several other studies; that middle school girls had higher FCAT math tests than those that were not physically fit or physically active.

The study also found that participants with higher physical fitness levels were in school more often than those with lower equivalents. It's noted that a focus on physical fitness in middle school girls can lead to better school attendance, which in turn leads to better academic performance.

The concept of self-belief also correlates to academic performance. The individual's self-belief in math and reading were significantly related to related exam scores in both genders.

The GPAs of students in the physical fitness improvement zone were also significantly higher than those in the lower, unhealthy zone. Now, this study helps to confirm what we already know about physical fitness and its correlation to academics. In addition, it shows that the girls – especially who may be at risk of low self esteem – improved their self image greatly by increasing their physical fitness and activity.

In a similar study by Bass, Brown, Larson and Coleman, significant relationships between physical fitness and reading and math scores for both middle school girls and boys were found.

The study suggested, again, that the kids who were more physically fit were more likely to academically pass all their classes than the kids who were unfit and inactive.

In a televised interview on health and wellness, Dr. Marla Shapiro helps confirm the direct correlation between exercise and grades. Her important research shows the fact that, as so many public schools have moved away from exercise and after school activities, grades and self esteem have suffered – an issue that is not just limited to the United States.

It is a consensus statement from 24 different countries, that clearly states that, *"physical activity not only boosts the obvious that we think about physical health – cardio respiratory health – but brain power, academic health, self esteem and motivation. There are a lot of benefits that we honestly do not often think about when we think about exercise."*

Dr. Shapiro also adds that, *"we have a lot of evidence that shows that kids who exercise vigorously enjoy much better heart health and cardio respiratory health, and it decreases the risk of long-term, down-the-road, middle-age diseases such as diabetes, heart disease, hypertension, and so on. But part of the exciting research shows that it doesn't matter if it's moderate or vigorous, or even if it's just a little bit of exercise. It really does make a difference long term, in lots of the metabolic markers that we look at. And when it comes to boosting brainpower, we know that kids who exercise during the day, before school, during school or after school show immediate improvement in their academic performance. And for kids who exercise, generally we do see that it boosts intellect working directly at the level of the brain.*

When kids exercise we think about the payoff for them in terms of emotional and intellectual quotient – overall physical activity in terms of metabolic skills, intellectual skills, self esteem, team building. It's something that we need to get back to doing. Really encourage our kids, and recognize that it as equally important as sitting in the classroom."

To summarize – there are physical, mental and physiological benefits to exercise. As we can clearly see, there is almost nothing that exercise – even just a little bit – cannot help with. This is important to note, because time and time again, schools decrease or eliminate exercise programs. Likewise, parents let their kids spend hours and hours in front of a TV or on a computer screen, and don't let – or *make* – their kids go out to play. Then they wonder why these children end up overweight, out of shape, depressed, sad, lonely, isolated and afraid.

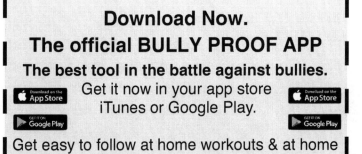

Make Physical Activity Part of Your Child's Life

Many physical activities fall under more than one category. This makes it possible for your child to do two or even three types of physical activity in one day!

For example, if your son is on a basketball team and practices with his teammates, he is not only doing vigorous-intensity aerobic activity, but also bone-strengthening. Or if your daughter takes martial arts lessons, she is not only doing vigorous-intensity aerobic activity but also muscle- and bone strengthening – plus she's getting bully proof. It's easy to fit each type of activity into your child's schedule; all it takes is being familiar with the following guidelines and finding activities that your child enjoys.

As a parent, you can help shape your child's attitudes and behaviors toward physical activity. Encourage young people to be physically active for one hour or more each day, with activities ranging from informal active play to organized sports.

Here are some great ways that you can do this:

- Set a positive example by leading an active lifestyle yourself. Martial arts is great for this, as families can train together to get fit and bully proof.

- Make physical activity part of your family's daily routine by taking family walks or playing active games together.

- Give your children equipment that encourages physical activity.

- Take young people to places where they can be active, such as your closest martial arts studio, public park, community baseball field or basketball court.

- Be positive about the physical activities in which your child participates, and encourage them to be interested in new activities.

- Make physical activity fun. Fun activities can be anything your child enjoys, either structured or non-structured. The Martial arts provides a cool way for kids to stay active while maintaining a healthy lifestyle. Other activities can range from team sports or individual sports to recreational activities such as walking, running, skating, bicycling, swimming, playground activities or free-time play.

- Instead of watching television after dinner, encourage your child to find fun activities to do alone or with friends and family, such as walking, playing chase or riding bikes.

- Be safe! Always provide protective equipment such as helmets, wrist pads or kneepads, and ensure that the activity is age-appropriate.

- Again, fitness programs such as KICKNFIT KIDS that include martial arts help kids feel comfortable in a positive, uplifting environment.

Find out more by visiting us on facebook:

https://www.facebook.com/bullyprooffitness Or Instagram: https://www.instagram.com/bullyprooffitness/

Bullying Happens to Adults Too

As tens of thousands of grown-ups already know, the cycle of bullying doesn't always stop in school. It can continue into your adult years, and even in the workplace.

From a definition used in the 2014 WBI U.S. Workplace Bullying Survey:

*Workplace Bullying is repeated, health-harming mistreatment of one or more persons (the targets) by one or more perpetrators. It is **abusive conduct** that is*:

- Threatening, humiliating, or intimidating.
- Work interference – sabotage – which prevents work from getting done.
- Verbal abuse.

Workplace bullying is driven by a perpetrator's need to control the targeted individual(s).

- Is initiated by bullies who choose their targets, timing, location, and methods.
- Is a set of acts of commission (doing things to others) or omission (withholding resources from others)
- Requires consequences for the targeted individual
- Escalates to involve others who side with the bully, either voluntarily or through coercion.
- Undermines legitimate business interests when bullies' personal agendas take precedence over work itself.
- Is akin to domestic violence at work, where the abuser is on the payroll.

Euphemisms intended to trivialize bullying and its impact on bullied people: Incivility, Disrespect, Difficult People, Personality Conflict, Negative Conduct.

Avoiding the word bullying where this behavior is concerned, in order to avoid offending the sensibilities of those who made the bullying possible, is a disservice to bullied individuals whose jobs, careers, and health have been threatened as the result. Tom Engelhardt explained it wisely when he said, "words denied mean analyses not offered, things not grasped, surprise not registered, strangeness not taken in, all of which means that terrible mistakes are repeated, wounding ways of acting in the world never seriously reconsidered. The words' absence chains you to the present, to what's accepted and acceptable."

In an article from Christine Comaford for Forbes.com, she wrote about how common workplace bullying really is and how much it takes a toll on businesses – both small and large.

Research from Dr. Judy Blando (University of Phoenix) has proven that almost 75% of employees surveyed had been affected by workplace bullying, whether as a target or a witness. *75%!* That's staggering.

So, what exactly is workplace bullying? According to The Workplace Bullying Institute, "workplace bullying is repeated, health-harming mistreatment of one or more persons (the targets) by one or more perpetrators. It is *abusive* conduct that is: threatening, humiliating, or intimidating, or work-interference, i.e. sabotage, which prevents work from getting done."

One of the main differences between schoolyard bullying and workplace bullying is that the latter tends to be less physically harmful and more psychological and verbal in nature. It may be more subtle than schoolyard bullying, but is quite distinctive from normal workplace stress.

According to a study by the WBI (www.workplacebullying.org), bullying is characterized by:

- Repetition (occurs regularly)
- Duration (is enduring)
- Escalation (increasing aggression)
- Power disparity (the target lacks the power to successfully defend them self)
- Attributed intent" (from Wikipedia)

Furthermore, according to the WBI, bullying is four times more common than either sexual harassment or racial discrimination on the job.

But who are these workplace bullies?

Here is what you have to understand – **the targets of workplace bullying are not always the weakest players.** In fact, they are sometimes the strongest. The common misconception is that, like schoolyard bullying, the targets of workplace bullying are loners – the people that don't fit in and are dubbed oddballs. In fact, the reverse is true.

People become targets because something about them is *threatening* to the bully. Often they are more skilled, more technically proficient, have a higher IQ, or people just like them better.

The bully often works hard to create the perception that they are strong by putting down and blaming others. Oftentimes, the boss of the bully knows the bully is disliked but thinks that the organization cannot do without them and makes allowances for their behavior. The bullying is framed as a personality conflict; a mislabeling that is costly in terms of time and money

From a 2007 survey of over 7,000 workers

- 37% of workers have been bullied: 13% currently and 24% previously.
- Most bullies are bosses (72%).
- More perpetrators are men (60%) than women (40%).
- Most targets (57%) are women.
- Women bullies target women (71%); men target men (54%).
- Bullying is four times more prevalent than illegal discriminatory harassment.
- 62% of employers ignore the problem.
- 45% of Targets suffer stress-related health problems.
- 40% of bullied individuals never tell their employers.
- Only 3% of bullied adults file lawsuits.

So, 37% of the U.S. workforce – that's an estimated 54 million Americans – report being bullied at work, while an additional 12% witness it. That is a total of 49% of workers. Conversely, 45% report neither experiencing nor witnessing bullying. Hence, workplace bullying is a *silent epidemic*.

A Different Kind of Harassment

Bullying is four times more common than harassment (based on illegal discrimination). Only one in five (20%) incidents of bullying result in discriminatory conduct.

Bullying Damages Employees' Health

The mythology surrounding bullying is that the targets complain and litigate frequently. However, 45% of targets experience stress-related health problems. Research from the WBI in 2003 found that targeted individuals suffer debilitating anxiety, panic attacks, clinical depression (39%), and even post-traumatic stress (PTSD, 30% of women; 21% of men). In addition, once targeted, a person has a 64% chance of losing their job for no reason. Despite the harm to their health, 40% never report their bullying.

How to Deal with Workplace Bullying

There are risks and costs to action. But they are far less than the long range risks of comfortable inaction.

- **President John F. Kennedy.**

If you feel like any of these things are happening to you at work, or to a colleague within your workplace, take these action steps. They may be scary or make you nervous, but consider the consequences of inaction.

Step 1. Report it. Tell HR, your superiors, or anyone that may have the power to stop the undesired behavior. Do not keep it to yourself, or pretend it's an isolated incident.

Step 2. Confront the bully by telling him/ her to stop – or try a snappy comeback from www.ishouldhavesaid.net such as:

• Too bad you can't Photoshop your ugly personality.

• Thank you for your brilliant portrayal of a self centered a@@hole in the movie of my life.

• You should really come with a warning label.

• I'm sorry I hurt your feelings when I called you a sociopath. I thought you already knew.

Step 3. Train, exercise, work out, build confidence in yourself and do something each and every day that's *just for you*. In the coming chapters, you will find out why this is so important – especially for parents.

15 Epic Reasons to Exercise

As you can see in study after study on kids and adults, *self-esteem rises when we exercise.* Test scores rise when kids exercise. Work gets better and more positive when adults exercise. Bullying decreases when we exercise. People of all ages not only look better; they *feel* better and they become smarter, safer and more self-assured than ever.

However, it's normal to have days where you just don't feel like exercising. You feel too busy, too stressed and quite simply too tired – and as a result, you forget about all the amazing benefits that a consistent and challenging exercise routine gives you and your whole family.

So, in case you need more motivation, here are fifteen of our top reasons to exercise. Pull out this list and read it to yourself or your kids when you're having one of those days.

1. **To Be Happier**

   Exercise has been shown to stimulate brain chemicals that induce relaxation and happiness, called endorphins. When you're having a bad day, lace up your shoes for an invigorating workout and feel happier.

2. **To Reduce Disease**

   Exercise has been proven to reduce the risk of pretty much every single health problem known to man, from stroke to heart disease, from cancer to osteoporosis. Exercise is also a great defense against Type 2 Diabetes, one of the most widely growing diseases of our time.

3. **To Look Amazing**

Exercise firms your muscles, improves your posture and even makes your skin glow. Looking amazing is a wonderful result of regular exercise. It's very rewarding when the people in your life start to notice your transformation.

4. **To Reach Your Goal Weight**

Exercise burns fat and helps you keep it off. If you want to have a leaner, healthier body, exercise is the answer.

5. **To Be Energized**

Remember that feeling you experience after a great workout? You're body is buzzing with energy, you're less easily irritated, and you feel more peaceful.

6. **To Get Better Sleep**

Exercise boosts energy levels during the day, but also wears you out. Recovering from a challenging workout will help you relax and reach a deeper level of sleep.

7. **To Slow Aging**

Regular exercise is one of the most effective ways to slow aging. When you age your body loses muscle and bone, and the loss of both are drastically reduced with regular exercise. You'll also enjoy a reduction in inflammation.

8. **To Reduce Back Pain**

   In most cases, the most effective thing that you can do for back pain is to move and strengthen those muscles. Always consult your physician or physical therapist for guidance if you have an injury.

9. **To Reduce Depression**

   Studies have shown that exercise is able to reduce depression – sometimes even as effectively as medication. Even if you don't feel like getting up off the couch to sweat through a workout, remember that you'll feel happier and more alive once you've done it.

10. **To Feel Fewer Aches and Pains**

    When you strengthen the muscles around your damaged joints you're able to reduce joint pain and overall aches. Remember to always consult your physician before starting an exercise program, especially if you have chronic joint pain.

11. **To Improve Memory**

    Exercise has been proven to improve memory and other cognitive functions, and seems to have a protective effect against dementia. A Harvard University researcher has been quoted as calling exercise, "Miracle-Gro for the brain."

12. **To Enjoy Your Life**

    Whatever it is that you love in life – your kids, travel, sports, fashion - it is all more enjoyable when you experience it in a fit and healthy body. Find the motivation to exercise so that you're able to enjoy all the great things in your life.

13. To Have Fewer Sick Days

Studies have shown that people who exercise regularly are 50% less likely to call in sick to work. With a regular exercise program you'll experience a reduced number of colds and upper respiratory infections.

14. To Burn Calories at Rest

Building your muscles through exercise means that you'll be burning extra calories even while at rest. You'll be able to eat more and maintain your ideal weight with ease.

15. To Be Confident

When you are fit, feel healthy and have energy, the natural result is great confidence. There's no better confidence booster than sticking with a regular exercise program. The results are more than worth your efforts.

Regular exercise gives you so many amazing benefits, which lead to a happier, healthier life. Get started TODAY

5 Reasons Why You Are Not Losing Weight

"The secret of change is to focus all of your energy, not on fighting the old, but on building the new."

- Socrates

Weight loss is often a frustrating pursuit, eluding even those who eat healthily and exercise regularly. So what gives? Why won't the scale budge, even as you put in tremendous effort? It's time to build new, *better* habits.

Read on for the 5 reasons why most kids and adults who exercise still don't lose the pounds that they want to…

1. **You Don't Sleep Enough**

   Let's start with the most rampant problem standing in the way of your fat loss; most adults simply do not get adequate sleep to support weight loss. There is a scientific reason for this, and it has everything to do with hormone levels.

   While you sleep, your cortisol levels decline while your growth hormone levels increase. This balance is essential for fat loss to occur. So skipping on Zzzz's will throw your hormones into fat-storing mode, while simultaneously causing you to feel hungrier and encouraging you to eat more calories.

2. **You Don't Drink Enough Water**

Most of us are walking around in a state of partial dehydration every day. In addition to being dangerous for all of your major body organs, dehydration is perilous for fat loss. Not only does water serve as an appetite suppressant to fill your stomach and prevent you from overeating, thirst is often mistaken for hunger pangs, leading to extra calories consumed and stored as fat.

By sipping on water throughout the day, you'll avoid dehydration and find it easier to move the number on your scale in a favorable direction.

3. **You Eat Out Too Much**

Restaurant meals are higher in calories than meals prepared and eaten at home – across the board. There is simply no way around it, and even if you consciously attempted to eat small portions while eating out, it would be quite difficult to do.

Restaurant food is created with consumer satisfaction in mind, and this means adding fats and sugars and salt to many of the menu items in order to produce the tastiest food possible!

Unfortunately the tastiest is also quite often the most fattening. Want more fat loss? In the coming chapters we give you the tips and tricks you need.

4. **You Don't Get Enough Protein or Fiber**

   Protein and fiber are the golden tickets to fat loss, but sadly your diet doesn't contain nearly enough of it. It's natural to enjoy the flavors of sugar, fat and carbs more than protein and fiber, and that's why your diet is filled with more of these than it should be.

   While sugar, fat and carbs taste better than protein and fiber, these lead to dreaded weight gain. Consciously plan your meals around a base of protein and fiber, and then add in just enough complex carbs and healthy fats to keep it well rounded. Save the bulk of your sugar, fat and simple carb consumption for planned cheat meals in order to prevent ongoing weight gain.

5. **Your Diet is Filled with Packaged Foods**

   I'm not talking about cookies and candies, because you know better than that. I'm talking about packaged granola, crackers, rice cakes, protein cookies, and the plethora of packaged health foods that you have stashes of.

   Sure, these packaged foods may be healthier than snacks from a vending machine, but in the grand scheme of your fat loss, the fewer packaged items the better when it comes to shedding pounds. Even the healthiest of packaged foods contain ingredients that are modified or processed, in order to preserve the shelf life and these ingredients have a negative impact on your waistline.

Real, natural and whole always beats packaged. Take inventory of your daily diet and eliminate the packaged foods so that it's no longer an everyday occurrence.

However, there is one most important reason that you are not losing weight – **you are not consistent**.

Ouch, right? Yes that may hurt, but you know it's true. One week you start eating healthily, you get the kids eating healthy, and you're all exercising daily. Then, by day four, you've found a myriad of reasons to quit. A few weeks go by, a few pounds creep on, and then you give it another try…for eight days this time before you quit. And the frustrating cycle continues.

The stunning body transformation that you want for yourself and your family will only come by changing your lifestyle as it relates to how you eat and how you exercise. Half-hearted attempts to change will only result in half-hearted results.Fully commit yourself to the process of transforming your body. Jump in with both feet and don't look back! As Socrates said, "stop fighting the old and start anew".

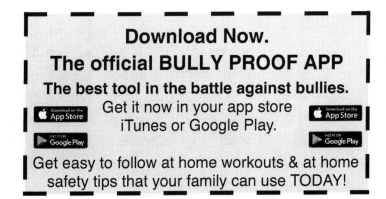

The Wake Up Call

Warning – this chapter is not for the easily offended. However, it is designed to help you and your family out of an unhelpful mindset.

One of the most popular questions we are asked is, "how do I get my kids to do this program?" The answer is simple – lead by example.

If you are a parent reading this book, you've got to get yourself in shape. If you are a coach, trainer, teacher or anyone in a position to influence kids, YOU HAVE TO GET IN SHAPE! No excuses, no baloney. You've got to start with *you*. And here's the great thing – this program was designed for kids to make them bully-proof and fit, but it will work for Parents, Aunts, Uncles… it'll work for anyone. Yes, even you.

The exercises in the **BULLY PROOF FITNESS** program are the same ones I do with my own kids, in addition to the thousands of kids I've helped throughout my career. **BULLY PROOF FITNESS** is interactive, fun and challenging at the same time, and the moves can be done almost anywhere, anytime. There are not many things that you can do as a family that are physically moving and fun. This program is the exception to that rule.

So, Mom and Dad… it starts with you. Your kids are inspired by you. You are their hero, their rock, their light. You are the alpha and the omega to those children. Whether you have one kid or five or a classroom full of kids, it doesn't matter. Get yourself physically fit and active.

And the other thing to remember – and this will be a common theme throughout the book – is that no matter what exercise you do, no matter what self-defense moves, no matter what physical thing I teach you, the number one takeaway that you need to know is you **cannot out-train a bad diet**.

You can work out seven days a week for an hour a day, but if you put the wrong fuel in your tank you are simply going to spin your wheels and fail to gain the results that you desire. If you don't get results, you get frustrated. And if *you* get frustrated, your kids will too.

You are the Super Soaker and they are the sponge. The more information, energy and lifestyle that flows out of you will flow into them. Then they will be more able to absorb it, and of course, the more fun it will be for your entire family. So, no excuses and no bullshit. It starts and ends with you whether you are in the position of parent, teacher, coach, administrator, manager, owner or leader. Be the living example of what you teach!

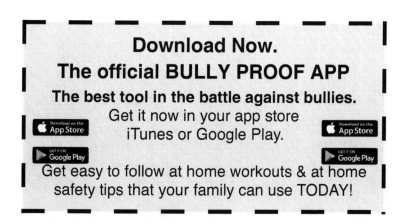

On the following pages you're going to see the secrets and tips of how we do **BULLY PROOF FITNESS**, but ultimately, everything that happens is based upon leading by example. Even if you've got a bad relationship with your kids, if you start doing this, you can help get your whole family right back on track.

Why is this so important? Well, do you remember these old sayings? *"Don't do what I do. Do what I tell you to do."* And the perennial classic, *"Because I said so."* That's the wrong way to inspire, lead and parent. You need to lead by example. You've got to walk the walk, and you've got to talk the talk. You want your kids to be bully-proof and fit? You can't just yell at them, or pop in a video and tell them, "get up off the couch and be fit." You, as the parent or guardian, have got to actually physically do something with them. *Please.*

That is the best way; getting involved in what they do. Here is the honest truth – *the overwhelming majority of overweight and obese children come from parents who themselves are overweight or obese.*

If that is you, then your first reaction to that statement may be the biggest problem and danger kids face today – **Denial**.

Denial is when you create excuses and say things like, "he'll grow out of it" (they don't); "I'm not fat!" (you are); "My kids and I are just big-boned" (you're not – dinosaurs are big-boned); "I just can't get them to eat anything healthy" (stop buying junk); "we're just a *little* overweight" (more denial)

FYI - being just 5-10 pounds overweight can double your chances of heart disease, diabetes, high blood pressure and stroke! Want proof? Then maybe you'll believe the World Health Organization and The American Heart Association, who have this to say.

Diabetes – Obesity is considered one of the most significant factors in the development of insulin resistance, and insulin resistance can lead to Type 2 Diabetes. According to the World Health Organization, more than 90% of diabetes patients worldwide have Type 2 Diabetes. Being overweight or obese contributes to the development of diabetes by making cells more resistant to the effects of insulin. A weight loss of 15-20 pounds can help kids decrease their risk of developing Type 2 Diabetes.

Heart Disease – According to the American Heart Association, obesity is a major risk factor for developing coronary heart disease, which can lead to a heart attack or stroke. People who are overweight are at a greater risk of suffering a heart attack before the age of 45. **Obese adolescents have a greater chance of having a heart attack before the age of 35 than non-obese adolescents.** If kids are overweight, losing 10-15 pounds can reduce their risk of developing heart disease. If they exercise regularly, the risk of developing heart disease falls even more.

Cancer – A study by the American Heart Association found that being overweight increases your chances for developing cancer by 50 percent. Girls have a higher risk of developing cancer if they are more than 20 pounds overweight. Regular exercise and a weight loss of as little as 12 pounds can significantly decrease the risk.

And there's more…

Research Studies Showing the Benefits of Activity on Academics and Overcoming Life Challenges

<u>Physically Fit Kids Have Beefier Brain – University of Illinois</u>

The brains of physically fit kids look and function differently than their less-fit peers, with increased brain white matter contributing to higher-fit children outperforming their lower-fit peers on cognitive tasks in the classroom.

Source - www.sciencedaily.com/releases/2014/08/140819083429.htm

Key Points:

- More physically fit = more white matter in brain.
- More white matter is connected to faster and more efficient nerve activity.
- The study found throughout one's lifespan white matter can be associated with increased physical activity.

More physical activity improved school performance –

More physical activity is shown to improve school performance in Swedish study.

"Two hours of extra physical education each week doubled the odds that pupils achieve national learning goals," according to Thomas Linden, a scientist and neurologist of the Sahlgrenska Academy.

Source – www.sciencedaily.com/releases/2014/10/141014094753.htm

Key points:

- The main idea is physical activity improves school performance.

- Results were clearly shown to support the idea physical activity improves school performance.

12 minutes of exercise improves attention and reading comprehension in low-income adolescents, as well as reducing stress levels.

A Dartmouth study shows that 12 minutes of exercise improves attention and reading comprehension in low-income adolescents, as well as reducing stress levels. The recommendation is for low-income school populations to incorporate brief bouts of exercise into their daily routine.

Source – www.sciencedaily.com/releases/2014/06/140612104952.htm

- Low-income group experienced a much bigger jump. This may be due to their higher stress levels.

- Improves selective visual attention among children as well.

- Actual Improvement in academics and activity – attention and reading comprehension

Look, you bought this book for a reason.

Maybe it was to understand bullying, or how to stop your child (or yourself) from being bullied. It might have been to find out to get your kids (or yourself) get in better shape. Or how fitness relates to helping your kids get better grades. We can help you with all these things – but the one thing you have to do is accept the truth. When you do, things can, and will, get better fast.

If you are a parent of a child who is overweight and/or being bullied, it is your responsibly, obligation and duty as a caregiver to accept that things are possibly not as great as you wish they were. That maybe you messed up somewhere along the way. That acceptance will get you more results than denying or making excuses for anything that has or will happen. And this book will help you and your family get better, grow stronger and get more bully proof than ever before. It is a guide, a path and a proven system to a better lifestyle.

Step one is to accept responsibility and open up your mind so that we can change the previously-held notions that it's societies fault. It's not a blame game, it's a mindset shift that will allow you to accept responsibility for what has happened and permit you to change the behaviors, patterns and trends that lead kids to being overweight, out of shape and being bullied.

<u>Step two, and just as important</u> – ideas are great, but implementation is everything. You have to take *action*. Even small steps in the right direction will lead to massive, determined growth and change that will get you the results you desire. Change is constant. Our job is to get you to stop thinking and start doing. Want results? Take action and you will get them.

It is our mission, plan and purpose to help and empower 1,000,000 kids and their families. **To do that, we need your help.**

Accept that things aren't working.

Decide that you *want* to fix it.

Commit to the plan in this book and focus on the long-term success of your family's health and wellbeing.

Success will be yours.

THIS PROCESS WILL WORK FOR YOU AND NOW IT'S TIME WE START!

Remember, this process works only *when you implement it*!

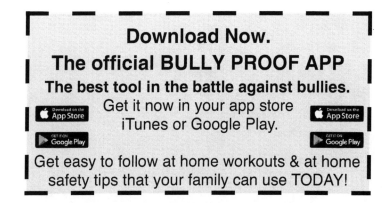

The Secret Formula for Bully Prevention

Our growing softness, our increasing lack of physical fitness, is a menace to our security.

- President John F. Kennedy

There are 3 steps to become bully proof and fit. Three easy steps than *can and will* change your life. We have seen this work thousands of times, and have watched it transform families just like yours for over 30 years.

1. Eat better

2. Exercise more

3. Rest

Rule #1 – You can't out train a bad diet

Said every health and fitness professional ever.

There is nothing more important than rule number 1. If you get nothing else out of this book other than food plans and eating strategies, you will be ahead of 75% of other people on this planet.

More than 10 million children suffer from obesity, considered one of the leading causes of life-threatening diseases. Being morbidly obese can compromise your health, shorten your life, and even cause death. If you are overweight, the probabilities of developing heart disease, diabetes, and high blood pressure increase significantly.

Food is Fuel – use it properly

The heart and soul of our **BULLY PROOF FITNESS** program is food and the proper fueling of the body. To understand how important eating the proper food is, let's take a look at **NASCAR®**. The high performance race cars used in those races are super-strong, very fast, and highly efficient. For these cars to operate at their peak they require a team of engineers, operators, mechanics and crew chiefs all working together to achieve the ultimate goal of winning the race.

However, if they forget to put the proper fuel in the car – a fuel that is a high-performance special mix – their car goes nowhere. Even if they put regular gasoline in the tank, the kind we use for our everyday vehicles, the racecar sputters, starts, stops and eventually just breaks down.

The kids (and you as the parent) are the high performance car, and *we* are the crew chiefs.

Your family is not going to go on a 'diet'. **We don't believe in diets**, because they are short-term fix to a long-term problem. Diets tend to work during their term, but if they are not sustainable they stop working.

We are going to teach, show and guide you on how to eat smarter and develop healthy eating habits that can be used all the time – even when eating out. The **BULLY PROOF FITNESS** plan is unique because once your family gets into the habit of eating correctly, you will all keep the weight off. Designed by a fitness nutritional expert, our eating plan sets up a balanced and common sense approach to good eating habits. A key point, and a fun one, of our eating plan is the six days on, one day off approach. This way your whole family can have a day to splurge if they want.

The BULLY PROOF
Food Planner

TIPS & POINTERS

1. This is *not* a diet! It is a healthy eating lifestyle, the choice of bully proof kids and star athletes.

2. You may substitute any type of fruit for another (e.g. Kiwi instead of apple, etc.).

3. No mayonnaise, *ever*, on anything. There are plenty of other condiment options for veggies and salads – all veggie dishes can be spiced up with salsa, ketchup, Tabasco®, garlic, or tomato sauce.

4. When eating out (option 1), order 2-3 appetizers and *share* – forget the entrées.

5. When eating out (option 2), order no appetizers, just the entree. When it arrives, box half of it to go!

6. When you prepare your meat, *no frying*. Bake it, sear it, grill it, or steam it.

7. Make the smart choices. Drink bottled water, or 100% real juice.

8. You must exercise *at least* three days a week for a minimum of 30 minutes – or else!

9. Junk food is exactly that – junk! We don't need it, and you *can* live without it. **Be disciplined!**

10. Focus on success! Nothing worthwhile was ever gained without sacrifice. It took time to put the weight on, and it will take time to see results.

The BULLY PROOF Shopping List

This shopping list goes with the meal plans on the following pages.

Juice
- ☐ Premium Water
- ☐ Simply Orange Juice w/Calcium
- ☐ Tropicana Pure Premium
- ☐ V8 juice

Breads *(No white or enriched White flour)*
- ☐ Ezekiel Bread any flavor
- ☐ Whole grain Wheat bread
- ☐ Whole Wheat English muffin
- ☐ Whole Wheat Pita Bread

Cereals
- ☐ Honey Nut Cheerios
- ☐ Raisin Bran
- ☐ Smart Start
- ☐ Special "K"
- ☐ Total
- ☐ Steel Cut Oatmeal

Snacks
- ☐ Balance Bars
- ☐ Cliff Bars
- ☐ Kids Z Bars
- ☐ MOJO Protein Bars
- ☐ Odwalla Bars
- ☐ Applesauce
- ☐ Turkey Jerky (low sodium)
- ☐ Low fat Peanut butter

Condiments
☐ Honey
☐ Ketchup
☐ Tomato sauce
☐ Mustard regular or spicy
☐ Salsa
☐ Tabasco or Cholula

Dairy
☐ 2% skim milk
☐ Eggs
☐ Low-fat Cottage Cheese
☐ Non fat milk
☐ Unsalted butter

Meats
☐ Chicken breast (Skinless)
☐ Fish-Salmon or Tuna
☐ Flank steak
☐ Ground turkey

Fruits & Vegetables
☐ Apple
☐ Asparagus
☐ Bananas
☐ Broccoli
☐ Carrots
☐ Celery
☐ Grapes
☐ Kiwi
☐ Oranges
☐ Raisins
☐ Strawberries
☐ Tomato

Breakfast	Snack	Lunch	Snack	Dinner
DAY 1 2 eggs scrambled mix with ½ cup low-fat cottage cheese, 1 piece-wheat toast	Non-fat or Greek Yogurt any flavor	4-oz chicken, ½ cup brown rice, ¾ cup veggies.	1 apple, banana, or any other fruit	4-oz fish, 1 cup pasta in garlic or tomato sauce, ¾ cup steamed veggies.
DAY 2 1 bowl cereal w low fat milk & 1 handful raisins or grapes	1 serving Turkey Jerky	1 tuna sandwich on wheat bread or pita- w/ no fat Mayo 7 carrot/ celery sticks	1 Protein Bar or 1 cup unsalted Mixed nuts	4-oz Flank Steak, ½ cup brown rice, ¾ cup steamed veggies.

DAY 3 1 bowl cereal & 1 cup grapes or strawberries	Non-fat or Greek yogurt any flavor	Chicken breast sandwich, w/ tomato, 1 slice low-fat cheese	1 apple, banana, or any other fruit	4-oz chicken breast or fish, ½ cup low fat cottage cheese
DAY 4 Hot oatmeal w/ ½ tablespoon low fat peanut butter, 1 handful raisins	1 apple, banana, or any other fruit	4-oz chicken breast, ½ cup low fat cottage cheese, & tomato	1 Protein Bar	4-oz chicken or fish, green salad, tomatoes, honey mustard dressing & corn on the cob.
DAY 5 2-3 egg whites, ½ cup apple sauce, 2 strips bacon 1 piece wheat toast	1 Protein Bar or 1 Greek yogurt	Turkey sandwich w/no fat Mayo, ¾ cup veggie	1 serving Turkey Jerky	4-oz Flank Steak, ½ cup brown rice, ¾ cup assorted steamed veggies.

DAY 6	1 Protein Bar or 1 cup unsalted mixed nuts	4-oz sliced chicken, 1 cup pasta plain, 7 carrot/ celery sticks	1 Protein Bar or 1 Greek yogurt	4-oz turkey burger on wheat bun, salad & honey mustard dressing.
1 bowl cereal w/ low fat milk & 1 whole banana				
DAY 7 **Off day** Eat what you want.	**Off day** Eat what you want.	**Off day** Eat what you want.	**Off day** Eat what you want.	**Off day** Eat what you want.

NOTE – all meals and snacks should include a 12oz glass of water

The Top 30 Fat-Burning Super Foods

Here is a great list to help turbocharge your metabolism so your family burns even more fat, and faster.

1. **Avocado**. It's rich in L-Carnitine that can help metabolize fat cells.

2. **Green tea**. Contains an antioxidant that boosts metabolism.

3. **Blueberries**. They contain soluble fiber to help you feel fuller for longer.

4. **Almonds**. They contain zinc and vitamin B to help curb cravings for sugar.

5. **Grapefruit**. Known to help boost metabolism.

6. **Oatmeal**. Contains soluble fiber that can also help you feel full longer.

7. **Salmon**. Includes protein to help build muscle for efficient fat burning.

8. **Flax seed**. Contains a high amount of dietary fiber, which is important for weight loss.

9. **Oranges**. They're high in fiber and help to curb your appetite.

10. **Tomatoes**. Contain 9 oxo-oda, a fat-burning compound.

11. **Apples**. Contain pectin, which limits the amount of fat your body absorbs.

12. **Hot peppers**. Help increase metabolism, speeding up the conversion of belly fat to energy.

13. **Olive oil**. Can fight off inflammatory diseases, including obesity.

14. **Raw apple cider vinegar**. Helps digestion and regulate blood glucose levels.

15. **Cinnamon**. One tablespoon of cinnamon can help regulate blood sugars.

16. **Quinoa**. Contains the complete chain of amino acids, is protein-rich, and boasts high amounts of fiber.

17. **Pine nuts**. Contain compounds that suppress the appetite by working against the hunger hormone.

18. **Bananas**. Have high amounts of soluble fiber to help slow down digestion.

19. **Mushrooms**. Low in calories and fat, and contain potassium for improved blood pressure.

20. **Coconut oil**. Easily digested by the body and converted into energy.

21. **Sweet potato**. Low in calories but high in fiber.

22. **Eggs**. Contain healthy fats and good cholesterol, and are a good source of lean protein that can help burn fat throughout the day.

23. **Lentils**. High in fiber, helping you feel full for a long time.

24. **Greek yogurt**. Contains a higher amount of protein and less sugar than regular yogurt.

25. **Chicken breast**: High in quality protein, which helps you build lean muscle.

26. **Broccoli**. Low in calories but high in nutrients and fiber.

27. **Asparagus**. A natural diuretic, which can help rid the body of excess water.

28. **Kidney beans**. Rich in iron, potassium and magnesium.

29. **Goji berries**. Contain chromium, an important trace element for preserving lean muscle mass.

30. **Kale**. High amounts of antioxidants, which can fight off inflammatory diseases including obesity.

Two Great Products To Help You Reach Your Goals Faster

Generally speaking, people who lose weight but not body fat are getting active, and even working out, but probably not eating according to the fitness plan. The weight they lose is water weight, and will stop after the second or third week. **Nobody can reach their goals if they are eating poorly.** Here are two things we think will help you and your family to stay on track.

The first thing we recommend is a good, reliable scale – one that measures both body fat *and* weight. We particularly recommend the Tanita brand scale, which can be purchased at major sporting goods stores, Target or Walmart.

Plan to spend $45-150. This may make you wince, but it's an important piece of equipment for goals and tracking progress. This gives parents, educators and care givers a valuable tool in helping to encourage children to make healthy lifestyle choices.

Read on for the difference between body fat and body mass.

Body Fat Percentage is the proportion of fat to the total body weight. Body Fat Mass is the actual weight of fat in your body.

Body fat is essential for maintaining body temperature, cushioning joints and protecting internal organs.

The energy, or calories, that our body needs comes from what we eat and drink. Energy is burned through physical activity and general bodily functions. If you consume the same number of calories as you burn, all the calories are converted into energy. But if you consume more than you burn, excess calories are stored in fat cells. If this stored fat is not converted into energy later, it creates excess body fat.

Too much fat can damage your long-term health. Reducing excess levels of body fat has been shown to directly reduce the risk of certain conditions such as high blood pressure, heart disease, type 2 diabetes and certain cancers.

Too little body fat may lead to osteoporosis in later years, irregular periods in women, and possible infertility. It is important to check your body fat results on a regular basis.

The second thing we recommend are good quality jump ropes, one for each person in your family. A jump rope is light, easy to transport and can be used almost anywhere, anytime, by anyone. **The best fighters, trainers and athletes in the world jump rope**, as it is one of the best ways to shed pounds and build coordination, stamina and skill while you work up a sweat.

Maybe your vision of jumping rope is tripping about PE class with a beaded rope and a bunch of 12 year olds. We get it. We were there too. But if you haven't picked up a jump rope since, or you're just afraid of looking silly at the gym, the next pages contain a few great reasons why jumping rope is one of the very best exercises out there (and *much* cooler than you think).

We recommend going to www.buyjumpropes.net. Don't buy the cheapest rope you can find, but neither should you pick up the costliest – the mid-priced ropes work well, and can be adjusted for smaller kids. Good quality ropes can be purchased for less than 10 bucks! Check out these cool tips from our friends at jumpropes.net

#1 - Calorie Cooker

Very few exercises burn calories like jumping rope. Even jumping at a very moderate rate burns 10 to 16 calories a minute. Work your jump rope exercise into three 10-minute rounds and you're looking at burning off 480 calories in half an hour. According to *Science Daily*, 10 minutes of skipping rope is about equivalent to running an 8-minute-mile. There's a reason the American Heart Association created an entire movement around jumping rope (ever heard of Jump Rope for Heart?).

#2 - Build Agility & Quickness

Want to get lighter on your feet? Skip rope every day for a few minutes. When you jump rope on the balls of your feet, body connects with mind to make neural muscular adjustments that help keep you balanced. Essentially, skipping rope improves your balance and quickness/coordination by making your mind focus on your feet for sustained periods of time, even if you're not conscious of it. Boxers know this. Why do you think jumping rope is a favorite exercise for the best boxers in the world?

#3 - Increase Bone Density

The medium impact of jumping rope increases bone density, but isn't as hard on your joints as running because the impact of each jump is absorbed by both legs. In fact, according to Dr. Daniel W. Barry, a researcher who has studied the bones of the elderly and of athletes, the latest studies show simply jumping is one of the very best exercises for improving bone density.

#4 - It's Good for Your Brain

We know that exercise (even as little as 20 minutes) is good for the brain. But did you know that activities with both physical *and* mental demands (like slacklining, ballroom dancing or jumping rope) have higher impacts on cognitive functioning than exercise tasks alone (like the treadmill or stationary bike)? Turns out the very best workouts for brain health involve coordination, rhythm, and strategy. So the next time you're jumping rope, challenge yourself to try some tricks. Turns out they're really good for your brain.

#5 - Jump Rope Tech

We've come a long way from the beaded ropes of PE class. Modern fitness ropes come with ball-bearing handles, ultra-fast cables and easy sizing systems (and the color customization options are endless). New 'smart' jump ropes will count your jumps. The new beaded ropes can also be customized with your favorite color of ultra-light, unbreakable beads.

#6 - <u>Affordability</u>

Of all the fitness options out there, rope jumping is still one of the most affordable. Shoot, even runners need to fork it over for high-end shoes. But jump ropes? Even a top-of-the-line fitness jump rope is only $20. Very simple (but high quality) ropes can be purchased for as low as $3. And, depending on the surface you jump on, a rope should last you a while.

#7 - Pick a Style, and Own it

Speed jumping. Chinese wheel jumping. Double Dutch. Jumping rope while juggling a soccer ball. Or crazy freestyle jumping (see above). There's seemingly no end of ways to have fun with a jump rope.

#8 - Portable

How else to explain this... *You. Can. Jump. Rope. Anywhere.* We've seen videos of people jump roping on the beach, on top of mountains, on boats ... even in the dark. Unless you live in a hobbit hole, you can find space to jump rope.

Get to www.buyjumpropes.net and start getting bully proof and increasing your fitness today!

Exercise and Self Defense

Physical fitness is not only one of the most important key<u>s</u> to a healthy body, it is the basis of dynamic and creative intellectual activity.

- President John F. Kennedy

OK, now that we have the meal plan and shopping lists in place it's time to get active.

We are going to cover all the basics for fitness, safety, self-defense and bully prevention in this book.

But if you haven't already done so….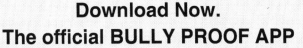

Bully Proof Workouts

"No man has the right to be an amateur in the matter of physical training. It is a shame for a man to grow old without seeing the beauty and strength of which his body is capable."

- Socrates

Before you begin any exercise program or a workout in general, the first thing to do is stretch. Stretching helps prevent injury, and warms the body up to prepare the muscles to work at their peak capacity.

Stretching

Ballistic stretching uses the momentum of a moving body or a limb in an attempt to force it beyond its normal range of motion. This is stretching, or warming up, by bouncing into (or out of) a stretched position, using the stretched muscles as a spring that pulls you out of the stretched position. This type of stretch is best reserved for advanced or professional athletes who are accustomed to training, working out and performing at their maximum capacity.

Static stretching means that a stretch is held in a challenging but comfortable position for a period of time, usually somewhere between 10 to 30 seconds. Static stretching is the most common form of stretching found in general fitness, and is considered safe and effective for improving overall flexibility.

With **BULLY PROOF FITNESS** we are going to focus primarily on _static stretching_. This type of stretching is best for beginners and intermediate levels, and allows people to appropriately warm up their bodies in order to help prevent injury.

Bully Proof Stretches

Here are two of my favorite warm-ups. Each warm-up and stretch should be done for 1-3 minutes – keep track using a timer on a cell phone or tablet to guide the routine.

☐ The Boxer Bounce

☐ The Seated (10) second stretch L, R, Center.

The Boxer Bounce

Unsurprisingly, this warm-up get its name from boxing. If you have ever seen a boxing match, martial arts sparring or an MMA fight you will know exactly what I'm talking about. It's a great warm-up as it engages the legs as well as the entire cardiovascular system.

To perform the boxer bounce; start with one foot slightly in front of the other, with your hands up in a defensive position and legs slightly flexed. Start your timer for 30 seconds then, staying on the balls of your feet, shift your weight from front leg to back in a gentle bouncing motion.

When you are performing the boxer bounce, try *not* to jump straight up and down – instead, bounce front to back in place, as though you were rocking in a chair. Keep your hands up in front of you like a shield, and remember to breathe with each bounce. When the timer beeps, switch to the other side without stopping.

Repeat this three times, then rest for one minute before proceeding to the next stretch.

The Seated 10-Second Stretch

Sit down on the floor, feet in front of you. This is a great stretch for the hamstrings (found on the back of your leg), the hip and the lower back. Take your legs and spread them apart as wide as you can, heels on the ground, toes pointed upward and legs straight. Sometimes, just the act of sitting in this position is difficult enough. Over time, you will gain flexibility and strength and your posture and position will improve.

BULLY PROOF TIP: BREATHE! The biggest mistake beginners make when stretching is holding their breath. This tightens up the muscles and prevents them from relaxing, which of course is the exact opposite thing we want to achieve. Take a deep breath and exhale slowly.

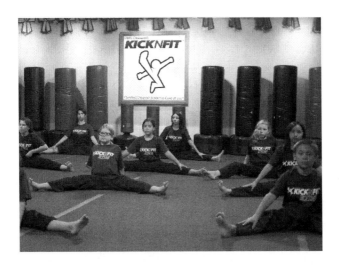

Once you are set in the proper position, take both hands and go forward as far as you can. Hold this position and slowly count to ten, allowing gravity to gently pull you forward.

After your count, slowly slide to your right leg with both hands extended and hold that position. Your goal is to have both hands touch the toes of your right foot, while keeping your leg straight. Slowly count to ten, then slowly slide to your left leg with both hands extended, holding that position.

Your goal, again, is to have both hands touch the toes of your left foot, while keeping your leg straight. Slowly count to ten.

Can't get very far? Knees bending as you move? Don't panic or worry – everything will be alright. One of the most wonderful things about the human body is its ability to adapt, learn and grow. Keep doing this stretch, and within a week or two you will see some amazing results.

BULLY PROOF TIP: Stretch twice a day. Once in the morning when you wake up, and again at night before bed. In the morning its gives your muscles a wake-up call, and at night it helps you relax from any kind of stressful day you might have had. Create the habit of stretching, and not only will you prevent injury you will grow stronger, leaner and more bully proof than ever before.

Super Kicks

There are dozens of kicks that come from a variety of styles of martial arts. Kicking is an important skill to learn because it helps develop balance, coordination, focus, accuracy and

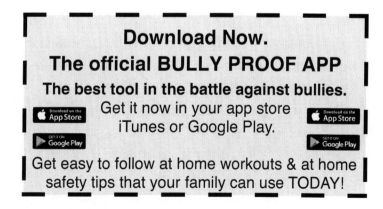

strength. Once perfected, it becomes a very effective style of self-defense and protection. This book will concentrate on the most efficient, and the fastest ones to master. For detailed instruction, and to continue developing your kicking skills – as well as punching and blocking…. Download the BULLY PROOF APP

The Front Kick

This kick is aptly named, as it is a move thrown straight forward. Start by taking a slightly staggered stance, with one foot slightly in front of the other. Place both hands up in front of the body and, using the rear leg, lift the knee upward. Extend the leg forward, or kick, and then return the knee back its starting position and placing your foot on the ground. Repeat this for kick for ten repetitions, then switch sides and use the other leg. The best athletes can kick effectively with both legs.

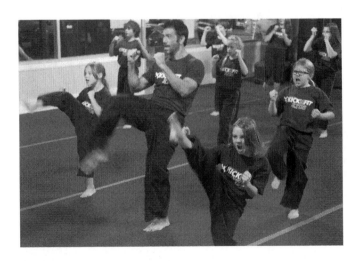

BULLY PROOF TIP: To be the best kicker possible, follow these simple rules:

- Keep your hands up and close to the body.
- Never swing the leg. Always lift the knee (chamber) first. This will make your kick faster and help to prevent injury.
- The leg you are standing on (aka your base leg) when kicking should remain slightly bent for balance. Don't rise up on your tippy-toes.

The Back Kick

Slightly more difficult than the front kick, the back kick requires more balance and coordination. This kick is also named after the direction it goes – backward, in this case.

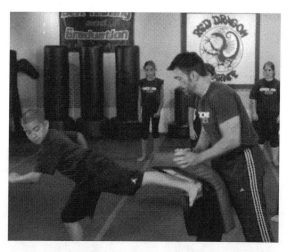

Start by taking a slightly staggered stance, with one foot slightly in front of the other. Place both hands up in front of the body, and using the *front* leg, lift the knee towards your belly. Look over your shoulder (same side) and extend the kick straight back behind you to complete the kick.

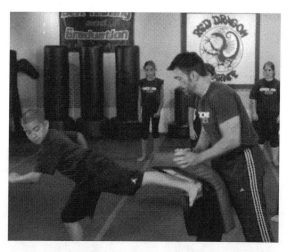

Bring the knee back to its starting position before placing your foot on the ground. Repeat this for kick for ten repetitions, then switch sides and use the other leg for ten more.

BULLY PROOF TIP: Don't try to kick higher than your waist. The back kick is meant to be low and strong. If you are bending your back or falling as you kick, try lowering the height until you build the skill and technique to go higher. But remember – **never give up!**

Awesome Strength Training

It goes without saying that there are hundreds – if not thousands – of strength training moves, and the variations of are endless. For this book we will stick with my personal favorite, and the ones that target all the major muscle groups. Plus it will help to provide a great full body workout.

The Push-Up
The push up may just be the perfect exercise to build both upper body and core strength. Done properly, it is a compound exercise that uses muscles in the chest, shoulders, triceps, back, abs and even the legs.

How to Do the Perfect Push-Up:

Get on the floor on all fours, positioning your hands slightly wider than your shoulders.Extend your legs back so that you are balanced on your hands and toes. Keep your body in a straight line from head to toe, without sagging in the middle or arching your back. You can also do these on your knees until you build the strength needed to hold your body straight through the entire push-up.

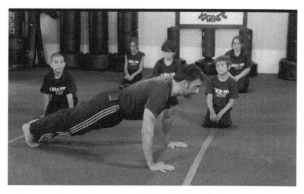

Before you begin the movement, contract your abs and tighten your core by pulling your belly button toward your spine. Keep a tight core throughout the entire push up.

Inhale as you slowly bend your elbows and lower yourself, until your elbows are at a 90-degree angle. Your body should be just an inch or two off the floor.

Exhale as you begin pushing back up through your hands to the starting position. Don't lock out the elbows; keep them slightly bent.

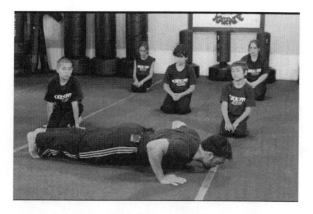

As you are working on mastering the push-up, focus first on form, then on quantity of repetitions. Just ten perfect push-ups a day (combined with the proper fuel as mentioned earlier) will lead to a stronger, leaner more toned physique.

Goal 1 – 10 perfect pushups.

Goal 2 – 30 seconds of non-stop push-ups

Goal 3 – 60 seconds of non-stop push-ups

BULLY PROOF TIP: The wider apart your hands are, the more challenging the push-up. For a basic push-up, your hands should be next to your chest, not in front of it, nor out past the width of your shoulders.

The Mountain Climber

Mountain climbers take their name from their resemblance to the techniques used to scale steep mountainsides. This bodyweight exercise is useful for burning calories, building stamina and strengthening the core. Not only do mountain climbers make use of all of the body's major muscle groups, they're simple enough to be done almost anywhere. When performed quickly, they're also effective as a form of cardiovascular training.

When doing the mountain climber you will build strength with the help of gravity. This exercise works the core muscles, quadriceps, hip flexors, and glutes, along with the chest, deltoids, lats, and lower back since they will be responsible for stabilizing the plank position.

How to do it

1. Get down on the floor on your hands and knees. Extend your legs out behind you, similar to the push-up position from earlier, balancing on the balls and toes of your feet. Place your hands directly under your shoulders with your fingers facing forward. Keep your core engaged by squeezing your stomach muscles. Your body should be in a straight line like a plank. Head up, hips in line with body.

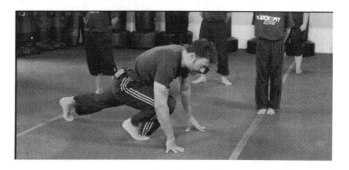

2. Pull one knee up and in toward your midsection, as though you are about to start running a race. Lift one foot and begin bending the knee as you pull it up between the front of your body and the floor. Bring the knee forward in one smooth motion. Don't let your knees sag or come into contact with the floor.

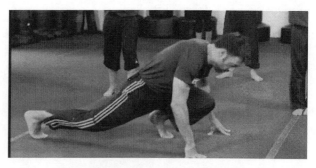

3. Repeat the action with your other knee. Relax your midsection and slowly push your knee back toward your other foot. Straighten your leg and set your foot back on the ground behind you. Then, bring the other knee forward, moving fluidly.

BULLY PROOF TIP: Don't allow your body to come out of alignment. A sagging rear end or V-shaped hip angle are symptoms of bad form. Hold your arms strong and straight, but don't lock your elbows.

Each up and back motion with your leg counts as one repetition, or rep.

Goal 1 – 20 reps.

Goal 2 – 30 seconds of non-stop mountain climbers.

Goal 3 – 60 seconds of non-stop mountain climbers.

5 Minutes a Day to Becoming Bully Proof and Fit

After you have taken some time to stretch and warm up, set a timer for 30 seconds. Perform each exercise and then move to the next – stopping only to reset the timer. After all the moves in the sequence have been completed, rest for one minute. Then repeat the circuit for the required rounds.

Combine this workout with the BULLY PROOF meal plan and you are on your way to SUCCESS!

A.   Boxer Bounce

B.   Front Kicks alternating legs (L&R)

C.   Push ups

D.   Back Kicks alternating legs (L&R)

E.   Mountain Climbers

Level 1 – Repeat this circuit twice (about 5 minutes)

Level 2 – Repeat 5 times (about 10 minutes)

Level 3 – Perform as many circuits as possible in 15 minutes.

Level 4 – Set the timer for one minute instead of 30 seconds, and perform the exercises in order as a circuit five times (about 30 minutes)

Self Defense

A common misconception people have about the martial arts is that they are designed to teach people how to be violent, and beat people up. Actually, quite the opposite is true.

Being in the Arts for the better part of forty years has allowed me to see, learn, experience and come to understand that the martial arts. In general, they were developed as a means of self-defense in order for people to be able to protect themselves from those who oppressed them.

The art of fighting and protection of self goes back thousands of years. Many people assume its origins are from Asia, but according to the history of the martial arts on Wikipedia, "the earliest evidence for specifics of martial arts as practiced in the past comes from depictions of fights, both in figurative art and in early literature, besides analysis of archaeological evidence, especially of weaponry. The oldest work of art depicting scenes of battle, dating back 3400 BCE, was the Ancient Egyptian paintings showing some form of struggle. Dating back to 3000 BC in Mesopotamia (Babylon), reliefs and the poems depicting struggle were found.

In Vietnam, drawings and sketches from 2879 BC describe certain ways of combat using sword, stick, bow, and spears."

For the purpose of **BULLY PROOF FITNESS**, we will focus on self-defense moves that are fast, efficient and easy to master – and work well for both kids and adults.

3 Pushes

Three pushes gets its name from the amount of moves, as well as the amount of times you will give a potential bully or attacker the opportunity to leave you alone.

Since we are teaching self-defense, and not self-*offense*, our first movement and technique will have us moving backward (away) from a potential attacker. When someone is approaching us and we do not know their intent or what they want we want to keep them out of our *Critical Distance Zone* (CDZ).

The CDZ is our safe area – to find yours, simply extend your arm straight out in front of you, fingers extended. The tip of your fingers is the CDZ.

When a stranger is approaching you, never allow them to be closer to you than this. No matter how fast or strong you think you are, when somebody is inside your CDZ your ability to protect yourself effectively decreases by 100%. There is a law of physics that states that *action is faster than reaction.* Therefore, their ability to strike or grabyou (the action) will always be faster than your ability to block or avoid it (your reaction) when they are inside your arm's length.

BULLY PROOF TIP: Through extended training, you will become aware of this zone without sticking your arm out in front of you. Since you would also look pretty silly walking around like that, practice with a friend or family member in the meantime. Have them approach you, and when they do tell them to STOP when you believe they are in the zone. Then, just lift your hand – if your fingers can touch them, you did it. Continuous training of the zone creates a hyper-sensitivity of the space around you, and gives almost 'Jedi'-like awareness.

Begin in a natural stance, feet about shoulder width apart. Place both hands up in a non-threatening manner; it should appear that you are raising your hands as though surrendering. The hands should be about as high as your head, not above. As they are approaching, take one step backward and ask, *loudly*, "what do you want?"

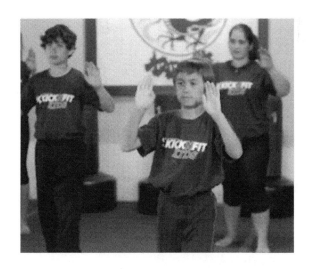

If they stop to answer, stand your ground, always remaining aware that they are *not* within your CDZ. If they continue to advance, take another step backward and announce, even louder this time, "I DON'T WANT ANY TROUBLE."

If they *still* continue to advance, take one final step backwards and firmly order (not ask!) then to STOP.

BULLY PROOF TIP: ALWAYS speak loudly - this takes practice. You can be, and probably *will* be, scared when confronted by a would-be bully or attacker. This human emotion (fear) is perfectly normal. It's OK to be scared, but it is *not* OK to *sound* scared. Be afraid on the inside. PRACTICE!

Moving backwards three times, and speaking loudly and clearly, communicates to the attacker – and anyone around you – that you are *not* the bully, that you *are* trying to protect yourself, and that you *do not* want to fight.

We limit our backward movement to only three steps for a few reasons, one of which is space. You may be in a parking lot, in a building, or in a space that doesn't allow you to back up without running into something behind you. In addition, you don't want the attacker to back you into an area with no people, and therefore nobody to possibly help.

BULLY PROOF TIP: Sad but true, many people aren't in the helping strangers business. When they see a possible threat, they may just keep walking and ignore it. With their faces in their phones, people are constantly caught up in their own augmented reality. That being said, if you need help, yell "FIRE!" Everyone wants to see a fire. Crazy but true.

If the attacker continues to advance towards you once you have exhausted the retreat and words, they are leaving you no choice but to defend yourself. From the hands up position, you will now execute the push block. This block is fantastic because it does not use force against force. This block allows a physically weaker opponent the ability to easily avoid a grab or a punch from a bigger, stronger attacker.

Move 1 – to properly perform the block, use the palm of the hand and push across your own body.

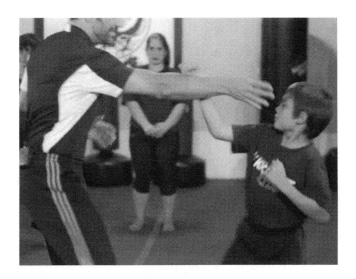

BULLY PROOF TIP: If you are right-handed, begin this three-move sequence with your right hand. Lefties, begin with the left hand.

Move 2 – as they approach again, or attempt to use one or both hands, take your opposite hand and push across your body with your palm leading the way.

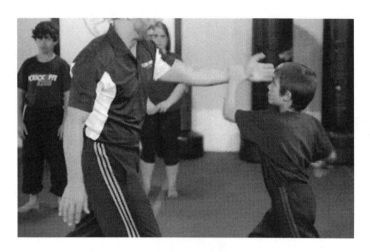

Move 3 – after you have blocked twice, you will finish with a strike we call the Palm Heel. This strike again allows a weaker defender to end the potential threat with one move. To properly execute a Palm Heel Strike, slightly bend the fingers of the striking hand and fold the thumb slightly inward. Push the bottom part of the palm (closest to the wrist) forward, and strike straight ahead while tensing the palm area.

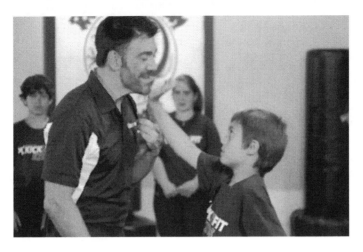

BULLY PROOF TIP: The Palm Heel strike is best thrown to the face, with the main target being the nose. The palm heel is a "one and done" move, so it is *not* a move to play with, only recommended as a last resort. We strongly recommend that you not only practice this move, but that you seek the help of professional instructors who can guide you through more detailed training in self defense. Find them at our website

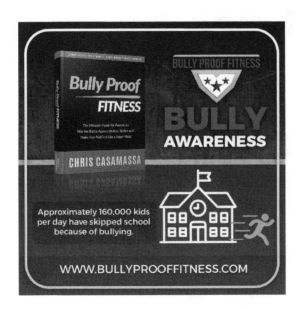

Bullying of Females

It can get worse!

Bullying isn't just about fighting. Women get attacked, abused and assaulted almost ten times more than men. Yes, you read that right – **ten times.**

Ladies, I'm sorry, but there are really are a bunch of bad guys out there. This is one of the reasons why I continue to do what I do. One of my goals is to train, teach and empower women to stand up for themselves, to fight the good fight, and to get them to know and believe they can survive an attack. How bad is it? Read on, starting with statistics and info from the Bureau of Justice.

The United States Bureau of Justice Statistics (BJS) is a federal government agency belonging to the U.S. Department of Justice and a principal agency of the U.S. Federal Statistical System. Established December 1979, the bureau collects, analyzes and publishes data relating to crime in the United States.

Rape cases during a 10-year-period were aggregated into a single data set consisting of 1,082 cases, which represent a national total of 1.5 million instances of rape or attempted rape. **Only about half the victims of rape or attempted rape surveyed stated that the crime had been reported to the police.**

Two-thirds of all rapes and rape attempts occurred at night, with the largest proportion occurring between 6 p.m. and midnight. Most victims of rape or attempted rape were white and young; the ages with the highest victimization rates for rape and attempted rape were 16 to 24. More than half of all victims had never been married, and most were members of low-income families.

The most frightening form of rape, an assault by a total stranger, was the most common. *More than 75 percent of all rapes involved one victim and one offender, and most offenders were unarmed.* Most victims offered some form of resistance. The most common responses to the situation were trying to get help; resisting physically; to threatening, arguing, or reasoning with the offender; or resisting without force. **The total cost of medical expenses reported was almost $72 million.**

The report also examines changes over time in the percentages of female victims of sexual violence who suffered an injury and received formal medical treatment, reported the victimization to the police, and received assistance from a victim service provider. Data are from the National Crime Victimization Survey (NCVS), which collects information on non-fatal crimes, reported and not reported to the police, against persons age 12 or older from a nationally representative sample of U.S. households.

MAIN FINDINGS:

- Between 2005-10, females who were aged 34 or younger, lived in lower income households, and lived in rural areas experienced some of the highest rates of sexual violence.

- Between 2005-10, the offender was armed with a gun, knife, or other weapon in 11% of rape or sexual assault victimizations.

- Between 2005-10, 78% of sexual violence involved an offender who was a family member, intimate partner, friend, or acquaintance During the past 25 years, a great deal has been learned about the psychological impact of rape.

The need for further research remains great, but it is pertinent to acknowledge the important role the Federal Government has played by supporting research programs on rape and other crime victim issues funded by the National Institute of Mental Health, the National Institute of Justice, and the National Institute on Drug Abuse (NIDA). The best data we have comes from the research funded by these agencies.

The research evidence shows that many rape victims sustain profound long-term psychological injuries. The research has found that a history of rape is a major risk factor for a host of major mental health disorders and problems. For example, when compared to non-victims, completed rape victims were 8.7 times more likely to have made a suicide attempt (19.2% vs 2.2%)

Sources: Kilpatrick, Best, Veronen, Amick, Villeponteaux, & Ruff.

Among women in the NIDA study, rape victims were over twice as likely as non-victims to have had a major depression (54.6% vs 21.9%) and they were 3.6 times more likely to have had major substance abuse problems (26.5% vs 7.3%).

Post-traumatic Stress Disorder (PTSD) is a debilitating mental health disorder that results from exposure to an extremely traumatic event such as military combat, natural disasters, or violent crime including rape. Data from the NIDA study indicated that over one-third (33.8%) of all rape victims developed PTSD sometime after their rape and that one victims in eight (12%) still had PTSD at the time they were assessed. Based on the estimate that **11.8 million adult women in the United States have been rape victims,** we can reasonably project that 3.9 million adult women have developed rape-related PTSD at some time, and that 1.4 million women in the United States have rape-related PTSD currently.

This suggests that the United States probably has more rape victims with PTSD than combat veterans with PTSD. It also suggests that many rape victims are not receiving effective mental health treatment for their rape-related mental health problems.

So, what now?

Women, please pay attention – for you, this is my #1 recommendation. **If you have a daughter, enroll her in the martial arts. If you are a female of any age, enroll yourself in a martial arts class, or kickboxing class. TODAY.**

I firmly believe that the martial arts, when properly instructed, not only build self-defense skills but also empower people (male and female) to be better versions of themselves.

After thousand of arrests, interviews and interrogations by police and FBI investigators, there was a common thread. Traits that attackers appeared to prey upon more often than anything else. *The victim appeared to lack confidence, had low self-esteem, or was generally unaware of their attackers presence.*

All these things can be fixed by becoming proficient in martial arts. Join a class now!

Rapist Beware

On the following pages you'll find excerpts from the book *Rapist Beware,* written by my father Louis D. Casamassa. He is a 10th degree Black Belt and the founder of our style of Martial Arts (Red Dragon), and he is also the creator of the Rapist Beware program.

My father started empowering women and training them to fight back in the 1980s. At that time, our main martial arts location was in the Southern California area. An area that was being terrorized by a serial rapist dubbed The Hillside Strangler – you may well have heard about him, I believe there was a movie. My father created this program in response to that threat, and even after Richard Ramirez was caught, tried and convicted, my father continued to teach and train women to fight back, grow stronger and survive. The United States Senate, Congress and countless local agencies have awarded him dozens of commendations and honors for his work with women.

WOMEN: THE WEAKER SEX?

From the book: Rapist Beware: by Louis D. Casamassa

All of their lives, girls and women have been told in one way or another that they are the weaker sex -- mentally and physically. And, it would appear, most women believe this. It has become programmed into women's subconscious minds in almost a subliminal way. When, as children, girls reach out to do things that men and society deem "unladylike," they are often labeled "tom boys," or worse – dike or butch. .

Most women are taught they can do nothing without a man. They are told: Marry a doctor; marry a lawyer; marry a man with a good trade, he will take care of you. This is programming at an early age. It makes women feel insecure and dependent on the men in her life. It can cause an inferiority complex, of which a woman may not even be aware.

Throughout history, of course, countless women in all cultures have demonstrated the fallacy in the notion that women are in any way inferior to men. The biggest change in American society has taken place since World War II,

especially in the economic sector. Today we see women occupying all sorts of positions formerly exclusively male: lawyers, doctors, police officers, truck drivers, heads of corporations.

As a woman, you must believe that you are physically and mentally the equal of men. Don't be patronized by men who say, "You've come along way, baby!" Say in return: "I have come a long way, and don't call me 'baby!"

This is not radical thinking. You must have this feeling through to your core. This is the attitude and thinking of someone who is equal.

You are the teachers of our children. Teach them from birth that men and women are equal, that women are not second-class citizens. In families where there are both boys and girls, never treat the boy as if he were better than or more special than the girl.

If you are a woman, think, for a moment, how strong you are. You give birth, a tremendous physical feat that requires a great inner strength. And each month, you endure the physical and emotional pain of menstruation, which can bring about a state of depression.

I suppose you might say: "Well, most men are bigger and stronger than I am." While this may be true, as a martial arts instructor, I know many small men who are stronger and faster than bigger men.

And I find it is much easier to teach women to fight than it is to teach men. Why? Women are natural fighters. It is natural for a female to scratch, bite, kick, pull hair, and rough-and-tumble roll around to just plain survive.

Here is a great story that my father would tell me about how strong and tough women can be, based on something that he saw and experienced first-hand during his time as a police officer.

When I was a police officer, one of the worst calls we could ever receive was a husband and wife fighting. And if we got a call about two women fighting, hell, we surely took our time getting to that situation!

I'll never forget a lesson I learned the hard way when I was a rookie. I got a disturbance call at a restaurant where two women were fighting. I was driving by myself on the west side of town, and I thought, Boy, this is going to be a breeze. I rushed to the scene, jumped out of the car and proceeded to break up these two pretty little ladies, when all of a sudden, Bam! Bang! Biff! Boom! It was like a scene from a Batman comic book. These ladies got insulted that a man was going to break up their fight! Forget it!

All I wound up doing was ducking -- fists, feet, fingernails, teeth, etc. I thought this was the end of my career as a cop, and remember, I'm a black belt in karate and judo.

Fortunately, assistance came, and I learned a real lesson -- not that you should respond slowly to women fighting, but that women can be strong, courageous and fierce in battle. The pain I felt in my arms from blocking blows was real, and no ess because a woman rather than a man caused it.

Even with two other officers, it took us a lot of time and great effort to subdue these two women.

So, ladies, please don't *ever* think that you are the weaker sex. The natural instincts women were given let you do something we have to *teach* a man to do, and that is survive.

Summary, Implementation and Action Steps:

My goal for you in this chapter is to motivate and inspire you to take action and help your family get bully proof and fit *now*. It's possible when you *take action and implement*.

I know this to be true because, after training and teaching thousand of kids and their parents and serving nearly 100,000 customers in over 35 years of full-time teaching, I have *seen* it work. I wish that I knew twenty years ago what I've shared with you in this short book.

I know it's not easy to get motivated, start, and change some bad habits while maintaining your health, sanity, marriage, relationship with your kids, staying balanced, happy and having a sound spiritual life.

But it's entirely possible to take a few shortcuts that can – and will – get you results. You'll lose weight faster, build more confidence and greater self-esteem, and get stronger without spending tons of time in a gym.

How? Just *start*. The sooner you start taking action and building momentum, the sooner you'll get stronger, lose more weight and be more confident.

If all you did was just got your kids or yourself to lose a few pounds, you are already a success. Momentum builds upon itself. It reminds me of a great quote, *"You don't have to be great to start, but you gotta start to be great."*

For small businesses such as gyms, martial arts studios, big box facilities, cross fit or boot camps, using our programs will allow you to gain new members, build more revenue and give back to the community you serve. Our programs are the pathways to profitability. Fast.

If you do have a company or business, and you are ready to get started implementing these strategies by having us teach or train your team with our award winning Rapist Beware program, KICKNFIT, or **BULLY PROOF FITNESS**, please go to www.chriscasamassa.com to get started.

I'm not telling you this to impress you, but to impress *upon* you how important getting started and staying motivated is – and it begins with getting into a mindset of belief.

In closing – I encourage you to drop me a message at rdkceo1@gmail.com, visit my website at www.chriscasamassa.com, and attend one of my free training webinars to help you build more confidence, lose more weight, get stronger, build a better lifestyle and stay on the path to fitness success all while becoming bully proof.

Get out there and implement, and keep me posted on your progress!

Chris

PS - be sure you visit me on <u>Facebook and post a comment or video about how much you like BULLY PROOF FITNESS, OK</u>?

About Chris Casamassa

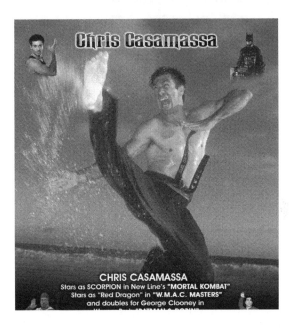

CHRIS CASAMASSA
Stars as SCORPION in New Line's "MORTAL KOMBAT"
Stars as "Red Dragon" in "W.M.A.C. MASTERS"
and doubles for George Clooney in

Originally from Bethlehem, PA, Chris moved to California in 1972 when he was just a small boy as his father wished to start a martial arts school in the warmth and sunshine of California, even though he had two successful locations in Pennsylvania. Chris trained side by side with his father from youth through adulthood, and as the Red Dragon company grew, Chris knew that he was destined to not only help his father run the studios but to take them from small time business to successful multi-unit operations.

For Chris, it's not all about the money - he's raised over $50,000 for the Make a Wish foundation and is on the board of the KID SMART FOUNDATION a non-profit charity whose sole purpose is to give back to underprivileged children in local communities by helping them cover tuition expenses to can train in the martial arts and become better, stronger adults that have developed leadership skills.

Chris has trained over 50,000 students (kids and adults) during the past 35 years in the Red Dragon studios, workshops, training seminars or at special events. He is a 9th degree Black Belt, and the current President of the fourteen Red Dragon Karate studios in southern California, where he directly oversees operations and helps studio owners grow their businesses.

With his core programs, KICKNFIT KIDS, The Kicknfit Challenge, B90Z Birthday party success systems and Lou Casamassa's Red Dragon Karate, Chris is grateful to be fortunate enough to have helped tens of thousands of martial artista, teachers and students achieve their goals.

Chris enjoys speaking, teaching, training and inspiring business owners, trainers, students and school owners around the globe on ways they can empower their students and supercharge their business.

He competed professionally on the North American Sport Karate Tour (NASKA) where he became a four-time national champion.
Chris has appeared in dozens of film and Television shows. Including *Batman & Robin*, *Walker: Texas Ranger*, *Buffy The Vampire Slayer* and many more. His signature role for his millions of fans around the world is Scorpion, the super-ninja from the hit *Mortal Kombat* films and TV series.

He lives in La Verne, CA with his wife Michelle and their children Emily and Adam – both of whom are bona fide fitness ninjas.

Chris can be contacted at his personal web site at www.chriscasamassa.com or through his social media channels.

Twitter – www.twitter.com/realmkscorpion
Facebook – www.facebook.com/chriscasamassa117 (fan page) and www.facebook.com/casamassa1 (personal page)

Book Chris Casamassa to Speak

Booking Chris Casamassa as your Keynote Speaker is a guarantee that your event will be inspirational, motivational, highly entertaining and unforgettable!

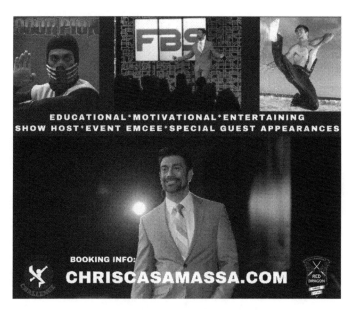

For over three decades, Chris Casamassa has been educating, entertaining, motivating and inspiring martial arts students, teachers and trainers, along with business owners, entrepreneurs, experts, consultants and coaches to build and grow their businesses with systems that are reliable, duplicatable and ones that produce consistent results.

After successfully helping over 300 business owners get amazing results with their business, Chris can share relevant, actionable strategies that anyone can use – even if they're starting from scratch.

His unique style inspires, empowers and entertains audiences while giving them the tools and strategies they need and want to get more members, provide better service, live a better lifestyle and continue to grow a successful sustainable business.

For more info and to book Chris for your next event, visit www.chriscasamassa.com

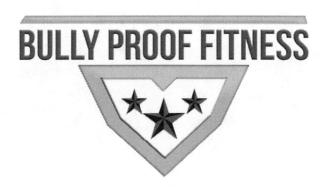

Made in the USA
Columbia, SC
21 August 2024

40861386R00061